BACK TO HEALTH

DR. FRED DIDOMENICO

Cover Design and Book Formatting by Vinnel Virgines

Edited by TMorgan Editing Services

In Collaboration with Legacy Creative
Library of Congress Cataloging-in-Publication Data:
DiDomenico, Fred
Back to Health / Fred DiDomenico
p. cm.

ISBN Hardcover: 978-1-637921-01-2
ISBN Softcover: 978-1-637920-95-4

1. Chiropractic. 2. Spinal Health. 3. Chiropractic Practice.
4. Spinal Subluxation.

Distributed globally by BeyondPublishing.net

www.elitecoachingllc.com

Table of Contents

Introduction
BACK TO HEALTH

Acknowledgments

...

I would like to acknowledge all the chiropractors that came before me, that paved the road we drive on. The chiropractors that were thrown in jail for adjusting sick people, the ones who fought prejudice and discrimination, the chiropractors that gave their lives for the principle of better health care advancing corrective techniques for a better life for humanity, too many to mention here. I give thanks to Dr. Don Harrison who gave his life to develop CBP technique, who passed it on to his son, Dr. Deed Harrison, one of the most highly decorated and published researchers in the history of the profession. Dr. Deed continues to give his life energy with his team of CBP doctors continuing to expand the research proving how spinal structure affects the spinal cord and nervous system breaking down health today. To all the medical doctors committed to research with clear and undeniable outcomes showing how distorted spinal structure can damage the spinal cord and cause disability, disease and even early death. To all those who give their life purpose for the betterment of humanity and the truth of optimal spine = optimal health, including all the patients who are living a better life in this lifestyle/better health decision. To God for creating all of us. Let's give back!

Introduction

...

Today's technology is weakening our bodily health. We injure and break down our spinal health as we bend over our smartphones to read or send text messages, play games, watch videos, or read notifications from our multiple apps. Even more, we slump at our computers for long hours, sit at the wheels of our cars, slouch at our desks, sleep on multiple pillows, and rest on the couch with our heads propped up watching our flat screens. This chronically forward-bending lifestyle is now known to break down our spines and may be ruining our health.

– Dr. Fred DiDomenico

This might sound alarmist, but it's true. While many people are aware that a sedentary lifestyle is not healthy, many people today—regardless of whether they live sedentary or active lifestyles, or anything in between—are adapting to a technology-focused way of living that can physically break down our bodies and cause pre-mature aging.

Technology is causing us to use our bodies in ways that put us into forward-flexed, head forward, shoulders rounded postures for prolonged periods of time that are changing our bodies and health for the worse. More and more teenagers and young adults are now showing up in doctors' offices with the kind of spinal degenerative disorders and health problems that in former times were only showing up in much older people.

Our bodies were not designed for this way of living. We are built to move. We're meant to use our strength, be dynamic and in motion. Movement helps our bodies heal injury and disease. Being in motion stimulates our brains. The normal, optimal structure of our spine and frame is designed to help us survive against the toughest of environments, the forces of gravity.

Our spine is the foundation of health and strength in our body. You will learn how a healthy, normal spinal structure allows life energy in the spinal cord to nourish all the organs with healing energy, giving us a stronger, more youthful body. You will also learn how the prolonged forward-bending postures can weaken and break down our spinal posture and structure, and how that causes premature degeneration of our spine and tension stress—like stretching a rubber band—to our spinal cord.

You will read research that details how this prolonged tension stress on the spinal cord can cause detrimental effects to our organs, including the lungs, heart, digestive tract, and more. This can also adversely affect our immune systems. If our immune system weakens, which is the system in our body that fights disease, you may experience anything from colds or flus to allergies, to autoimmune diseases, which can progress to cancer.

In addition, poor posture can lead to other, even more serious problems. With a distorted spinal structure causing increased sympathetic stress, overstimulation of the sympathetic nervous system leads to a decrease in the activity of the immune system with a resultant susceptibility to infection.[1]

Today, 8 out of 10 Americans have back pain, which means at least 80% of the population is suffering from unhealthy posture, which may or can potentially lead to disability and disease, and may even be life threatening.

---

[1] Stress, Immune function, and Health, the Connection 1999, Wiley-Liss Bruce Rabin pg 114.

I wrote *Back to Health* to bring awareness, choice, empowerment, and a plan of action to you, so that you and millions of others may live a better life. You have the choice to become aware that how you use your body and spine can determine both the quality and quantity of your health and life.

More than education, however, I'm offering you action steps to prevent this technology-overloaded effect on your posture and your spine. In fact, I have developed what I call the 5-10s, which I will go over in detail later in *Back to Health*. After ten minutes of poor posture (posture that's often technology-enabled), you can perform the four activities that I've designed that will temporarily relieve the stress and strain on your spine and spinal cord, and one that will make permanent change with the most effective, research-based spinal rehabilitative system to correct a weakened spinal structure.

These activities will affect your spinal structure, which, in turn, can help your bodily health. Structure determines function. A normal spinal structure determines your athletic performance with balance, coordination, symmetry of movement, better reflexes, increased circulation, more stamina, and greater endurance. Most important, normal spinal structure leads to confidence in the strength and health of your body now and in the future.

When I found this system and corrected my own spinal structure after I became a chiropractor, my health problems actually disappeared! These included degenerative, bulging discs resulting in weekly nerve pain in my arms and legs that had been troubling me for fifteen years. In correcting the structure, I also eliminated allergies, digestive issues, immune system problems, recurrent lung infections and continue to live the life of a healthy athlete today.

I have been given a gift of life, strength, health, and most importantly confidence and freedom. I want everyone else to have the same gift. For this reason, I have written this book and am speaking all over the world. This is a message for humanity. Start with you!

◇◇◇◇◇◇◇◇◇◇◇◇◇◇◇◇◇◇◇◇◇

BACK TO HEALTH

...

The ding cut through all other surrounding noises, like a razor-sharp ax spitting a piece of wood in one blow. He felt a rush of anticipation about what might appear, a hit of adrenaline to the bloodstream. Was it a text? Was it an exciting photo? Or a notification from one of his many apps?

Quickly, he reached into his pocket and pulled out his smart phone. He lowered his head, flexed his neck forward, and rounded his upper back into a relaxed, hunched posture as his fingers sped along the keys, translating thought into a message. He stayed in this position as unnoticed minutes flew by, immersed in multiple conversations, checking app notifications, and scrolling through seemingly endless posts, charging his curiosity.

Like many other people in this new technological world, he was addicted.

Aside from the many challenges of this technologically and emotionally charged lifestyle, the prolonged forward-bending and flexed postures that we subject our bodies to today can make us weak and unhealthy, ruining our physical health in ways most people are completely unaware of. Every day, our unconscious, prolonged, and repetitive physical habits drag down the strength and health of our bodies like an anchor.

But you can live a healthier, stronger, more empowered life that will not only help slow the rate at which you age, but will also enhance the quality of your life. You will find that knowledge here. And with that knowledge comes power. You will now have the power of conscious choice.

◇◇◇◇◇◇◇◇◇◇◇◇◇◇◇◇◇◇◇◇◇◇◇◇

OBSESSION BECOMES A SUBCONSCIOUS HABIT

. . .

O ur subconscious mind rules 95% to 99% of our life, according to Dr. Bruce Lipton, author of *Biology of Belief* and researcher at the Stanford University School of Medicine. This means that our conscious mind, the thoughts we're aware of, rules only 1% to 5% of our thoughts.

What's the significance of this? Our emotionally driven behaviors are neurologically "wired" into our brains and guide our actions. We're not always what we consciously think, nor are we always acting in ways that are driven by conscious intention. Often we're unaware of the automatic, reflexive actions we take, along with people and conditions we bring into our lives.

Many of our thoughts and behaviors originate from what has been programmed in our minds from our past, based on the "feelings" we experience and the decisions we have made at specific moments. Conditions that happen in our life become associated with and linked to an emotional state, and this pairing of conditions and emotion tends to stay neuro-emotionally coupled.

When similar conditions occur in our present and future, we re-experience a similar emotion that occurred in our past, and we take a predictable and repetitive action.

Have you ever wondered why you keep doing the same things or keep attracting the same people in your life?

Each condition may look different in the beginning, only for you to discover it may be very similar to a past experience.

This is the job of the limbic brain. The limbic brain deals with emotions, memories, and arousal (stimulation). It connects to our frontal lobe, our conscious mind—so we think we're acting with intention when, in truth, we're driven by our subconscious, pre-determined, emotional patterns.

This foundation of information is established in the beginning here because it relates to decisions we make on how we use our body and the short and long term effects on our health and life.

Thanks to the proliferation of such modern technology as smartphones, iPads, technology based games and more, we now live in a very repetitively and spontaneously hyper-stimulated world. Clever, researched, intentional marketing and technology have driven our brains and bodies into an excited and stimulated frenzy.

While technology gives us many advantages, it may also contribute to our physical breakdown. Our technologically advancing world makes our lives easier when our devices work, but we are left with a feeling of almost complete, temporary powerlessness when they don't. Emotionally driven, variable reward, the next unknown, anticipated adrenaline hit are what keep us immersed in the excitement of spontaneity repeating in succession.

Our brains neurologically adapt to our feelings of excitement with the next text, picture, video, or alert. In addition to these programmed reactions, we also have six basic, innate needs as humans. Anthony Robbins discusses these in his teachings. He based them on Maslow's Hierarchy of Needs. Adam Sicinski also talks about them in an article on *IQ Matrix*:

> *The Six Human Needs are not desires or wants. They are psychological "needs" that we constantly work to satisfy on a mostly unconscious level of awareness. These Six Human Needs are the factors that influence your deepest motivations and effectively determine how you go about prioritizing your decisions and actions throughout your life. In fact, every single day of your life you are unconsciously striving to meet these "needs" with varied success.* [2]

[2] Sicinski, A. Six Human Needs. IQ Matrix. http://blog.iqmatrix.com/six-human-needs

THESE SIX HUMAN NEEDS ARE:

1. Certainty: The need to ensure that you have comfort and predictability on some level. This minimizes the fear of the unknown.

2. Uncertainty: This is the need for variety and spontaneity, to relieve boredom, predictability, and stagnation, as life is motion.

3. Significance: This is the need to feel important with yourself and in the eyes of others. This need can create a sense of self-identity.

4. Love and Connection: We all need to be connected to people and in relationships. We also need to feel loved, to give love, and to belong.

5. Growth: We have a need to continue to learn and grow mentally, emotionally, and spiritually, in a variety of ways.

6. Contribution: We need to give and add value to something greater than ourselves.

Most people focus on meeting at least two of these needs that drive much of their behavior. For instance, someone whose primary need is significance might immerse himself in a career and strive to achieve success because that's tied to his identity and self-worth. Or a person may use his career to contribute to the lives of others to fulfill the need of contribution.

Another person may have a primary need of certainty and feel she must control every aspect of her life or else she is stressed and anxious. That second need, uncertainty, drives their fear.

When your behavior meets three or more needs, there's addiction. This is one of the reasons it is so difficult to stop an addiction; it satisfies deeply seated emotional needs for that person. This is also why logic has no influence to change addicted behavioral patterns. They are emotionally driven on a deeply rooted level that satisfies subconscious, perceived "needs," even though they may be destructive.

Technology, combined with hard-to-shake apps, meets three or more needs for many people.

For example, Facebook provides connection with other people by allowing you to follow them, view their posts, or see the posts they recommend. It provides certainty that it will be there, which satisfies certainty.

It satisfies uncertainty because you never know exactly what post will pop up next, so you scroll down from post to post. Facebook gives you significance because anyone can post a selfie, or talk about what they ate for breakfast, share what they did on a Tuesday night, or just describe how they feel in a moment. Some people may contribute a positive-mindset quote, as a reminder to themselves or others. So there are at least four needs being met, and, therefore, the potential of an addiction being created.

In his book *Hooked* (2014), Nir Eyal describes the qualities of subconscious habit-forming products and services. First is the Trigger, a psychological stimulus that leads to two, Action, which is initiated from a Trigger. Then, three, comes Variable Reward, the next uncertain stimulus, followed by four, Investment—the time or money you invest to engage in an action.

You may be asking yourself, "I thought this was a book on back health? Why all this information on marketing and addiction?"

Here's the connection: an emotional addiction to technology can injure and weaken our bodily health. We put ourselves into prolonged, flexed, hunched-over postures. We shift our heads forward toward our chests. We bend our necks and curve forward. We round our shoulders. We curve our backs into a hump. We put pressure and stress on our whole spine and nervous system. All of this distorts our spinal structure and places us in a structurally and biomechanically weakened position.

The diagram below shows how our body begins to flex forward when we use our cellphones and how a 10-pound head creates the load and force of a 60-pound bowling ball that could possibly collapse our spine.

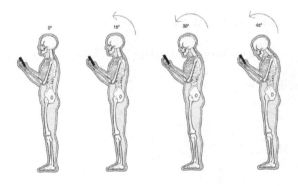

More importantly, this causes stress to our spinal cord, the lifeline of our body, which may affect the conduction of energy to our body's vital organs. This is a posture that may affect your health and well being right now!

We sit at our computers, live on our smart phones, drive in our cars, sit at our desks, sleep on multiple pillows. We lie with our heads propped up on a couch and watch our flat-screen TVs. We live our lives in prolonged flexion, forward-bending activities and postures that promote a spinal alignment associated with chronic pain, disability, pre-mature aging, cardio and pulmonary disease, and even premature death.[2] This book will show you the astounding, compelling, and awakening research showing you how we live our lives today setting us up for disability and disease.

[2]   Ozer, E., Yucesoy, K., Yurstever, C., Secil, M. (2007). Kyphosis One Level Above the Cervical Disc Disease: Is the kyphosis Cause or Effect? Journal of Spinal Disorders & Techniques, 20:1, pp. 14-19. Departments of Neurosurgery and Radiology, Dokuz Eylul University: Izmir, Turkey.

◇◇◇◇◇◇◇◇◇◇◇◇◇◇◇◇◇◇◇◇◇◇◇◇

WHAT'S NORMAL?

⋰

The lifestyle we have created is not the lifestyle for which our bodies were created and designed. Our bodies are meant to move, to have strength to carry out tasks, and to have a strong structure to resist the prolonged forces of gravity. Movement helps our bodies heal injury and disease, and stimulates our brains and grows our intellect. Our spines are the foundation of health, life, and strength in our bodies. Our spinal column keeps us upright. It's the foundation of muscular strength and neurological function. The spine also protects the spinal cord that carries life energy from the brain to and from every cell and organ in our body for its function.

The normal and optimal spinal structure is very specific and extremely important.

When looking at the spine, the structure should be straight from front to back. From the side, it should have three curves, as the following image shows. The spinal structure encourages us strength and health.

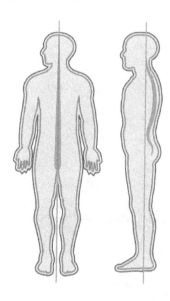

Dr. Don Harrison, founder of Chiropractic BioPhysics®, has researched and documented optimal spinal structure with his team.[3] He and his team have found that any deviation from this normal structure leads to breakdown of the spinal structure, stress and tension to the spinal cord, and breakdown of overall health.

---

3   Evaluation of the assumptions used to derive an ideal cervical spine model, Journal of Manipulative and Physiological Therapeutics, Volume 20 Number 4 may 1997, Donald D. Harrison, D.C., Jan J Janik, PhD., Stephen J. Tryanovich, D.C., Deed E. Harrison, D.C. and Christopher J. Colloca, D.C.

          Elliptical Modeling of the Sagittal Lumbar Lordosis and Segmental Rotation Angles as a Method to Discriminate Between Normal and Low Back Patients, Journal of Spinal Disorders, Volume 11, No 5, 1998. Donald D. Harrison, Rene Cailliet, Tadeusz J. Janik, Stephen J. Troyanovich, Deed E. Harrison, Burt Holland.

          Can the Thoracic Kyphosis be Modeled with a Simple Geometric Shape? The result of Circular and Elliptical Modeling in 80 Asymptomatic Patients, Journal of Spinal Disorders and Techniques, Vol 15, No.3, pp 213-230, Deed E. Harrison, Tadeusz J. Janik, Donald D. Harrison, Rene Cailliet and Stacy F. Harmon.

From a strictly biomechanical perspective, the normal spinal structure is strong and can withstand compression forces of running, jumping, and motion. It also provides the muscular strength and leverage for power. The straight-line structure from the front keeps the body aligned and in a plane-line of optimum strength. This is like hammering a straight nail into a board. A linear structure is strong.

The normal spinal structure should have three curves from the side. They are not equal curves. The cervical spine (neck) represents a piece of a circular arc. The thoracic (mid-back) spine is a piece of an ellipse, like the curve of an egg. An egg is not circular, yet it is strong when you try to push the ends together. The lumbar spine (lower back) is also in the shape of an ellipse, like an egg. These specifically designed structures allow the spine to distribute the constant compressive forces of gravity when we are upright.

That means no single segment or vertebra of the spine absorbs all the force as our bodies contend with the constant compression force of Earth's gravity. With its three curves from the side view, the spine acts like a spring, absorbing the effects of compression from running, jumping, walking, carrying objects, and other activities.

When the spine has this normal, healthy, strong structure, force is transmitted throughout the whole spine with far less chance of injury or weakness. Most importantly, the spinal cord will be relaxed and healthy, and will transmit healing energy, like a firehose, to all the organs of the body. A healthy spinal structure allows for a healthy, well-functioning spinal cord, thus allowing life energy to transmit to your organs, encouraging optimal health and strength. The result is you will enhance your ability to live a stronger, more confident, youth-filled life.

◇◇◇◇◇◇◇◇◇◇◇◇◇◇◇◇◇◇◇◇◇

Structure and Function

...

T he muscles that attach to the spine also have a mechanical advantage and more leverage for maximum strength when they can pull from or to the normal strong spinal curves.

The spine is a foundational structure that gives the muscles stability and strength to pull from to create motion. For the muscles to attach, insert, and ultimately to properly function, the normal spinal structure should be straight or vertically erect from the front, while from the side there must be three normal curves for maximum contractile strength, stamina, and power in all movement. When these curves are present, you are physically stronger and stable—your muscles feel less stress and tension and are more at ease.

This means your muscles are more relaxed when they are at rest and not required for full contraction. Therefore, they have more energy and more power when you do need them. When you lose the optimal spinal structure from chronic poor posture, sports, or other types of injuries, or if for some reason your spine never developed a healthy, strong structure, your muscles lose the proper leverage to work effectively.

As a result muscle contractions will be weaker and the muscles will work much harder to support and create movement when the spine, the structural foundation for strength, is weakened due to a distorted structure. The muscles now have a significant biomechanical disadvantage. Basically, your overall body strength can become weaker and more tired, with less stamina and endurance, more muscle spasms, and greater susceptibility to injury. This could be one reason people get weaker as they get older and the strength of their core—their spine—distorts and degenerates.

Structure determines function. A normal spinal structure enhances your athletic performance with balance, coordination, symmetry of movement, better reflexes, increased circulation, more stamina, and greater endurance. You'll have more powerful muscular contractions and increased overall performance.

A proper spinal structure leads to an optimally functioning nervous system, which provides the electrical power for the muscles. This is also why almost all professional athletes today are under regular chiropractic care. If many professional athletes use chiropractic for maximum performance, is it good enough for you?

With an optimal spinal structure and properly functioning nervous system, the muscles function more efficiently. You will have more energy available for normal physiological function, like healing, metabolism, and building your immune system, thus preventing disease.

◇◇◇◇◇◇◇◇◇◇◇◇◇◇◇◇◇◇◇◇

Neurological Function

...

L et's talk more about spinal structure and its effect on the spinal cord.
As I mentioned earlier, the spine houses the spinal cord, the
extension and connection of the brain that delivers life-force energy
in the form of electrical energy impulses to every organ in the body. The spinal
cord is our lifeline. It's the direct connection from our brain into our body. The
nerve tracks oriented in specific locations in the spinal cord bring energy for
specific functions in the body. Every function of the body depends on that nerve
energy to give it life and healing. With 100% energy, there's health. With 0%
energy, there's death. It's very simple.

Problems begin when the spinal structure is weak or distorted—and especially when stuck in a hunched, forward-flexed posture, which leads to a progressively worsening, degenerative condition from stress and tension on the spinal cord. Since the spinal cord is encased within the spinal structure for protection, it is subject to mechanical forces of stress and strain from a distorted spinal structure. When there is mechanical stress on the cord the healing energy in the cord diminishes, therefore, life energy keeping your organs healthy cannot be delivered to your organs.[4] Anything less than 100% energy begins the process of progressive disease. The weaker and more malaligned the structure, the faster you will degenerate, age, and suffer with more disease. It's a straightforward concept.[5]

The following chart shows the nerves that send strength and energy to the muscles, which are voluntary. This means that you are aware of moving your arm, and your brain uses these nerves to execute your intention. The nerves that bring energy into your extremities also control sensation (what you feel). Circulation (blood flow) is in this nerve distribution as well.

---

[4] Breig, A, El-Nadl, AF; Biomechanics of cervical spinal cord: Relief contact pressure on overstretching on the cord. Acta Radiol Diag (Stockh) 4:602-624, 1966.

[5] Wolff's Law reference: http://www.oxfordreference.com/view/10.1093/oi/authority.20110803124341929

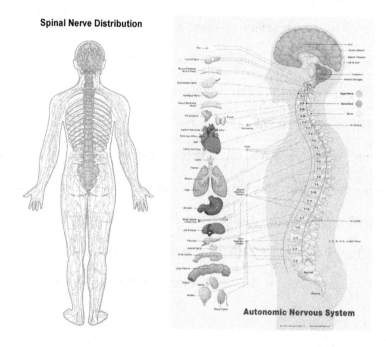

Spinal Nerve Distribution

Autonomic Nervous System

The sample chart on the right is the autonomic nervous system, the system that controls automatic function, such as the beating of your heart, the movement of your lungs, your digestion, and other bodily actions that you don't consciously think about. All of these functions are controlled by and depend on a healthy nervous system.

The spinal structure has a direct impact on the energy flow—electrical impulses—to every organ in your body through the spinal cord. When you have a strong spinal structure with normal curves, as I described earlier, your spinal cord is very relaxed, the diameter of the cord is thicker, and energy flows very easily and rapidly, delivering healing life energy to every organ in your body, like a cable from a power source, or a firehose.

Some nerves have impulses surging through the spinal cord at 390 feet per second. If you close your eyes and move your arms, you automatically know their physical position because the nerves for this muscle motion travel at this speed.

Touch travels at 350 feet per second.

Pain nerve fibers move much more slowly. For example, when you stub your toe, nerve impulses travel at 250 feet per second. That's why you won't feel the full pain for a second or two.

All these functions are transmitted through the spinal cord.

Reflexes are direct neurological paths from the spinal cord back to motor nerves in a quick loop. They don't need to travel to the brain. For example, when you touch something really hot, you move your hand away almost faster than you can think. This is a shorter neurological loop without the brain's more time-consuming interpretation, which is an important protective mechanism.

All other messages travel through the spinal cord to and from the brain to direct your physiology, or they're sent to the brain from the body through the spinal cord. The brain interprets them in a feedback loop through the spinal cord again and then to the organ, tissue, or cell to direct optimal function.

For this to happen at its highest level, the spinal cord must be healthy, without physical stress. It must be free from tension, allowing energy to bring healing and optimal health to the body. The proper curves from the side and a straight-line structure from the front are essential for the spinal cord to be in a relaxed, freely flowing, healthy state.

◇◇◇◇◇◇◇◇◇◇◇◇◇◇◇◇◇◇◇◇

STRUCTURAL AND BIOMECHANICAL DISTORTION OF THE CURVES

...

The spinal structure can distort and develop abnormally from a variety of causes, sometimes even in the womb. Distortion can occur as a result of stressful positions in the womb. Many newborns suffer from kinematic imbalances due to suboccipital strain, which may lead to symptoms like, torticollis, unilateral face asymmetry, C-scoliosis, and motor asymmetries, often accompanied by unilateral maturation of the hip joints and slowed motor development.[6]

During delivery, "A majority of newborns suffer from micro-trauma

of brainstem tissues in the periventricular areas.... Consequently, the

motor development cannot develop normally.... Later on, at the age

[6] Kinematic imbalances due to suboccipital strain in newborns. Journal of Manual Medicine, June (No. 6) 1992, pp. 151-156. www.danmurphydc.com/wordpress/wp-content/uploads/archive/.../Article_32-04.pdf

of 5 or 6, they suffer from headaches, postural problems, or diffuse symptoms like sleep disorders, being unable to concentrate, etc.[7]

This type of trauma is also a known cause of Sudden Infant Death Syndrome (S.I.D.S.). A study of 695 infants showed that high cervical-mechanical irritation could serve as a trigger in sudden infant deaths.[8]

Cervical trauma can cause spinal structural development problems in children, including S-Curve deformity of the spinal structure from the front, which is known as scoliosis.

In truth, many of us as adults have been these children who were plagued with subluxations, misplaced vertebrae, or misplaced curves and regions of the spine, and who've never had these problems correct or, worse yet, were unaware. Right now, your children's spinal development may be determining their health for the rest of their lives. Be sure your child is developing a healthy spinal structure and nervous system from the beginning of life to ensure better health, strength, and life.

---

[7]   Biedermann, H. (1992). Kinematic Imbalances Due to Subocciptal Strain in Newborns. *Journal of Manual Medicine*, June, 6, pp. 151-156. The Surgical Department of the University of Witten-Herdecke: Witten-Herdecke, Germany.

[8]   Kocha, L.E., Kochb, H., Grauman-Brunte, S., Stolled, D., Ramirese, J.M., & Saternus, K.S. (2002). Heart rate changes in response to mechanical irritation of the high cervical spinal cord region in infants. Forensic Science International, 128:3, pp. 168-176.

During our formative years, most of us experienced childhood falls and seemingly mild, "normal" childhood injuries and sicknesses. We endured physical activities, sports, and injuries. We've been involved in automobile accidents, lifting injuries, slips, falls, and countless opportunities for poor postural habits.

All of these incidents, some seeming inconsequential and meaningless, were compounding. Some have traumatized our spine, even if they occurred without our conscious knowledge at that time. When you look back, you will also see how health problems followed certain traumas. For instance, there's often a decline in energy levels and an alteration of your immune system function, sometimes followed by bouts of allergies, colds, or the flu after cervical and upper-back trauma. Left uncorrected, many times these conditions progress into stomach and digestive problems. As spinal problems progress and grow, so too may health problems.

I was born with my umbilical cord around my neck, which was strangling me with each uterine contraction of my mother. I was an emergency C-Section. I was colicky as a baby. As a child, I had sinus problems, stomach aches, and headaches. I had a compromised immune system. I often suffered from colds, flu, and had mononucleosis in second grade. Although I was never diagnosed with a major disease, I grew up fighting different sicknesses. I had so many throat infections that I had my tonsils out when I was 23. When I became a chiropractor and corrected my spinal structure, all of my health problems resolved, including the degenerative, bulging discs and nerve pain in my arms and legs that had been troubling me weekly for 15 years.

During my 14 years of chiropractic practice, I have also had the privilege of correcting the spinal structure of thousands of kids and adults, leading to overall better health and a better life for most.

In the following illustration, you can see a distorted, injured spine. The lines represent the spinal structure within this posture. Since posture is a window to spinal structure, it also represents the areas of stress on the spinal cord inside the spine.

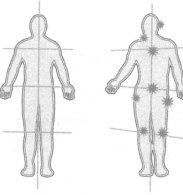

*Normal Spinal
Alignment*

*Weakened, Injured
Posture and Structure*

A distorted posture equals a distorted spine. A distorted spine negatively affects the vital life energy to the organs. In other words, as the spine twists, bends, and turns in its structure, the spinal cord, housed in your spine, also twists, bends, and turns. A person's health may begin to break down when stress on the spinal cord shuts down the energy to the organs.

◇◇◇◇◇◇◇◇◇◇◇◇◇◇◇◇◇◇◇◇◇

SUBLUXATION

...

When an individual bone is partially misplaced, this is called a "subluxation," a medical term for a displaced vertebra.

In fact, an individual subluxation–a single vertebra out of place–is less common than a whole section or region of the spine being "subluxated," or out of place from the normal structure, as seen in the previous illustration. We are not referring to an antiquated construct of a chiropractic subluxation. Instead, we are measuring a subluxation using validated, peer-reviewed, and published methods. Normal ranges of segmental and global alignment are well established.

Typically, an individually subluxated vertebra results from an extreme amount of biomechanical stress from the weakness of a whole curve being forced into one segment. As you can see from the diagram, to say a vertebra is out of place and only address that one vertebra without looking at that region and curves of the spine—and the whole spinal structure, in the majority of cases—is incomplete. It's more often the case that the spine as a whole is causing excessive stress on that vertebra and also may be related to a trauma. The detrimental health effects of a whole-spine problem could become severe. Unfortunately, many chiropractors focus on individual vertebrae without looking at whole curves. Again, the majority of times this is incomplete. As a patient you should ask to review the whole curves and regions of the spine compared to the normal structure on X-ray. Without X-rays, spinal structure, especially the curves from the side view, cannot be assessed accurately without X-rays. Any other "opinion" is just not true. Any other opinion is just not true and has not been validated in medical and chiropractic peer-reviewed literature. As such, I suggest you seek a chiropractor who has the training to apply a corrective treatment program. The doctor must analyze and then restore the normal curves and structure measured with a pre- and post-X-ray. This comparison side by side is essential.[9]

---

9   Lippa, L., Lippa, L., & Cacciola, F. (2017). Loss of Cervical Lordosis: What is the Prognosis? Journal of Craniovertebra Junction Spine, Jan-Mar 8(1), p. 9-14. doi: 10.4103/0974-8237.199877

⬦⬦⬦⬦⬦⬦⬦⬦⬦⬦⬦⬦⬦⬦⬦⬦⬦⬦

BACK PAIN

...

Eight out of ten Americans will experience back pain in their lives.[10] Back pain is the most common reason for all missed work days. Fully one-third of disability claims are related to lower-back pain.

Why is back pain so common? Because it's where the distortion in your spine becomes most evident. Your lower back supports your upper body, which is as much as two-thirds of your body weight and is the core strength of your body affecting your body's movements.

When your spine is distorted and weak, it collapses downward due to gravity. As a result the bottom of your spine—the lower back—is forced to bear the load of this collapsing spinal structure from above. Some may feel pain above their

---

[10]   Defrin. R., Benyamin, S., Aldubi, R., & Pick, C. (2005). Conservative Correction of Leg Length Discrepancies of 10 mm or Less for the Relief of Chronic Low Back Pain. Archives of Physical Medicine and Rehabilitation, November 86(11), p. 2075-2080.

lower back, such as neck and mid-back pain, and some may not. Obviously, most people feel pain in their lower backs.

The normal side view of the lower back is an ellipse, the curve of part of an egg. This gives the foundation of your spine its strength, like a spring or shock absorber.

When this curve changes, weakens, or distorts, the core strength in your body weakens. In other words, your whole body weakens. The discs become compressed form abnormal compressive forces of body weight and gravity—think of pressing onto one side of a water balloon—and, over time, that balloon with continual pressure can now burst as repetitive stress and compression weaken its outer fibers. This is similar to a herniated disc. Abnormal and asymmetrical compressive forces weaken the disc and cause it to bulge and eventually burst.

Structural corrective chiropractic intervention can help heal bulging discs, just like taking your hand off one side of a water balloon, depending on the severity of the injury. By correcting the spinal structure, relieving the abnormal biomechanical compressive forces on the disc always is a benefit at any point, especially if you've had surgery. People blow out discs because of abnormal biomechanics of the spine, whether it is caused by weakened and distorted posture over time or a sudden traumatic event. If the discs herniate–or burst like a water balloon–surgery may be indicated, however, many times corrective chiropractic has been very effective at reducing bulging discs, even after they herniate. Going to the right structural-corrective doctor and evaluating your condition is crucial.

Medical doctors today now know they must restore the normal curve before fusion surgery, or patients will continue to have poor outcomes. In fact, doctors have created the term, "Failed Back Surgery Syndrome" (FBSS), for post-laminectomy surgeries where patients received no relief or became worse after surgery. This typically results when when people did not correct their structure, so their disc problems and related symptoms returned or were never relieved with surgery.

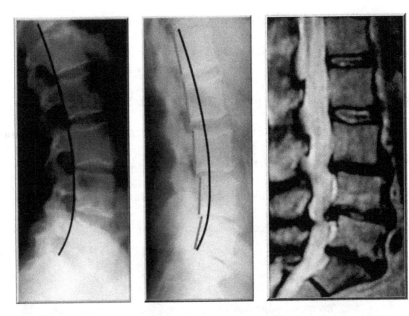

The photos show different views of the spine. The one on the left at the top shows a normal side view of a lumbar curve. The middle photo is an X-ray of a weakened, distorted structure with degenerated discs. The photo to the right is an MRI of the same patient, showing the result of disc compression bulging into the spinal cord.

These are the results of distortion and weakening of the spinal structure. Spinal-cord compression from direct impingement on the disc breaks down the function of the body at the level of the disc injury and below. A person with this condition may have numerous symptoms, such as pain in the legs, sensory and motor loss, bladder dysfunction, bowel dysfunction, sexual dysfunction, eventual disease in the pelvic organs and below, and more. This person is, or will be, disabled.

Studies show that many people with this type of injury may even be asymptomatic.[11] Research has found that between 35% and 75% of the adult American population has asymptomatic disc herniation. The renowned orthopedic surgeon Scott Boden, in a paper titled "Abnormal Magnetic-Resonance Scans of the Lumbar Spine in Asymptomatic Subjects: a Prospective Investigation," addressed this:

> *We performed magnetic resonance imaging on sixty-seven individuals who had never had low-back pain or sciatica. The scans were interpreted independently by three neuro-radiologists who had no knowledge about the presence or absence of clinical symptoms in the subjects. About one-third of the subjects were found to have a substantial abnormality.*[11]

When people with this type of condition casually bend over or do some sort of mundane daily task, they might suddenly become paralyzed by the sensation of a hot, sharp sword driven into their back unable to move. The pre-existing misalignment has probably been unknowingly present for years.

11   Spinal Compression Missouri. Asymptomatic Disc Herniations. Blog. http://www.spinaldecompressionmissouri.com/blog/asymptomatic-disc-herniations

There's a reason that you have pain or another problem with your back: it's been building up, regardless of whether the symptoms come and go. The reduction or resolution of the symptoms doesn't mean the underlying problem has been corrected. A weakened spinal structure only moves one way—progressively worse, even if the symptoms are not present.

There is only one way to know if a weakness in your spinal structure exists and that is through a series of upright X-rays combined with external digitalpostural assessment. You either have a normal structure or you don't. The only variable is the amount of distortion from normal. The further your spinal structure deviates from normal the weaker it is and the more stress is on the spinal cord affecting your health. The problem is many doctors may tell you that you have a spinal structure that's not the optimal structure and then tell you, "It's *your* normal," or it's not correctable. The truth is, it's not normal. It's common. Car crashes, heart attacks, and cancer are also common; however, they certainly aren't normal. The next truth is there is a system of spinal rehabilitation that can correct many or most of these problems we talk about later in this book. If eight out of ten people get back pain, then it's quite common. It's also leading people into chronic pain, disability, and disease. Our lifestyle today is making it worse.

If you tend to get yearly check-ups, would it make sense that you should get your whole spinal structure examined, X-rayed and be screened for possible weakness that may set you up for pain, disability, and disease? Consult a trained, structural-corrective doctor in Chiropractic BioPhysics®, which is the most advanced, researched, and evidence-based spinal-corrective system.

I include this because many people think their pain is in one area of the spine because that's what they feel. Can a person with full-body, metastatic cancer have pain in one area? That answer is yes! In this case, that one pain brings a person to a doctor, where they discover they are in a severe crisis with full-body metastasis.

Since our spine houses the spinal cord, which directs life energy to all the organs, it is important to check the whole spine, even when only one area hurts, because the whole spinal cord may be under stress and weakening your overall health. Is it smart to treat a localized area, or to look at the whole system for correction?

◇◇◇◇◇◇◇◇◇◇◇◇◇◇◇◇◇◇◇◇◇◇◇◇

Spinal Structure and Disease

...

In 1921, Henry Winsor, M.D., dissected 50 cadavers to determine the connection between abnormal minor curves in the spine and their relation to diseased organs. He concluded:

...in 50 cadavers with disease in 139 organs, there was found curve of the vertebrae, belonging to the same sympathetic (autonomic nerves) segments as the diseased organs 128 times, leaving an apparent discrepancy of 11, in which the vertebrae in curve belonged to an adjacent segment to that which should supply the diseased organs with sympathetic filaments...nerve filaments leaving the spinal cord and traveling for a few segments...where there were faint curves and slight visceral pathology.

In other words, 139 out of 139, for 100%.

The disease appears to precede old age and to cause it. The spine becomes stiff first and old age follows. Therefore, we may say a man is as old as his spine...[12]

Dr. Winsor found that where there were abnormal spinal curves, there were also diseased organs related to the nerve levels of those abnormal spinal curves. I cite this study because medicine has known this research since 1921. Why hasn't medicine told you? How many have suffered, even died, because of this "misinformation?" Would health care in this country be different if this was common knowledge?

The distortions in structure in the diagram seen on page 27 show a shift in whole regions of the spine. The red flares are areas of the body that will be suffering from abnormal compression loads breaking down the joints and leading to disability. These shifts in regions of the spine causing nerve and cord injury are related to diseased organs in Dr. Winsor's study. The picture of the spine in this diagram from the front and back may look extreme because the lines are clearly depicting the magnitude of the distortion.

---

[12] Medical Times (November 1921). The Evidence of the Association, In Dissected Cadavers, of Visceral Disease with Vertebral Deformities of the Same Sympathetic Segments. Medical Times, November 1921, pp. 1-7.

In reality many people walking around with this level of spinal and postural distortion and injury are only mildly aware of the extent of their problem. But a distortion of as little as 5 mm from optimum (or 0.196 of an inch) begins to create a significant weakness in the structure, causing it to progressively weaken and collapse. This seemingly minor distortion would not be detectable by a non-trained person, even missed by many professionals. For this reason, X-rays are imperative. With today's technology, radiation concerns associated with X-ray are a thing of the past, especially compared to the danger of missing this condition. There is no conclusive evidence of radiation causing harm at the levels patients receive from diagnostic X-ray exams.[13] The weaker and more distorted the structure, the faster and more rapidly it will degenerate and cause disease.

This becomes dangerous, because without this information, you yourself would probably not even notice a distortion of 5 or 10 mms visually in a mirror. In reality, if you or anyone can see a postural/spinal distortion on the outside, it is much worse on the inside. They would appear as one shoulder being higher than the other, one pant leg being longer, one sleeve on your shirts being longer, and abnormal or accentuated hump in your mid or upper back, your head tends to tilt to one side, you tend to stand a certain way with your hand on your hip or wear your purse on the same shoulder because wearing it on the other shoulder isn't

---

[13] https://hps.org/documents/meddiagimaging.pdf

comfortable. These are a few of many signs your spinal structure is weak, which may be affecting your health, energy, immune system and determining fast how your body ages.

Remember, the spinal cord is encased in that spinal structure. In every "kink" of the spine shown in the previous diagram, you can imagine a corresponding "kink" in the spinal cord.

This is an injury point to the cord that will cause direct neurological problems, since it may come into direct contact, causing pressure points on the cord as it rubs against the vertebrae. This inhibits the energy flow at that level of the spine to the associated organs, altering the function of the body. The part of the cord that has pressure and damage relates to the function of the body that becomes damaged and disabled.

The spinal cord will always take the path of least resistance. This principle is analogous to a car on a race track, hugging the inside corner of a turn in the track. The spinal cord will do the same, staying closest to the inside of the bend in the spine to avoid as much tension stress as possible. It moves closer to the inside edge of the bony spinal canal and will contact and chronically rub the bone on the inside edge side of the vertebral canal.

This rubbing causes pressure in the lateral corticospinal tract, the bundle of nerves traveling on the sides along the length of the cord, called a tract, controlling muscle function. Pressure on this tract may cause symptoms similar to Amyotrophic Lateral Sclerosis (ALS, which is sometimes referred to as Lou Gehrig's Disease). This is motor loss from degeneration of the motor tracts in the cord. This disease is believed to have an autoimmune origin—the immune system attacking the nerves. Multiple sclerosis is a similar type of disorder, an autoimmune disease.

The word "sclerosis" means the abnormal hardening of tissue of the body. It's like a callus on your hand from repetitive use or pressure, like working with your hands or commonly from weightlifting. You also have calluses on your feet from walking barefoot. Calluses form from constant contact and physical stress.

The spinal cord will develop an area of "sclerosis" when it has been subjected to long-term friction against the bony canal of the vertebrae and spinal column when your posture and spinal curves are weakened and distorted. In other words, the spinal cord will develop a callus.

This sclerotic area—blocks the nerve impulse like a dam in a river, and stops the electrical impulse. Wherever in the body that nerve tract carries energy will lose function. The lateral tracts—motor tracts on the side of the cord—will lose function, and will be classified as sclerotic diseases. In these diseases and situations, the muscles are not getting the nourishment (electrical impulses) they need, because the lateral cord has a callus, a type of friction rub. Prolonged friction will harden the tissue. This is the sclerotic area of a spinal cord that is in prolonged contact and friction with the vertebral canal.

This is one cause of these diseases, even if this is not the identified cause or official diagnosis. It is important to know that most diagnoses name the symptom, not what's causing it. The name of a symptom does not tell you what to do about it to correct it. Medicine tends to give you a medication to calm the symptom after the assigned name, yet may not directly handle the cause. With this strategy, you feel better while your body continues to get sick because the cause may not have been addressed.

Poor posture creates a weakened immune system through increased nerve and spinal cord stress. I wonder if anyone has ever checked the spinal structure of ALS and MS patients?

In the Journal of Vertebral Subluxation Research, August 2, 2004, Dr. Erin Elster published a study of 44 multiple sclerosis (MS) patients and 37 patients suffering from Parkinson's disease (PD). In all 81 cases, upper cervical (the top vertebrae in the neck) injuries were found. The study says that after trained chiropractors administered treatment to those upper cervical injuries, "44 (91%) MS cases and 34 of 37 (92%) PD cases showed symptomatic improvement to care, with symptoms improved and/or reversed and no further progression of either MS or PD detected." This study is not published in the premier medical research journals, yet the patient results remain. Although more studies need to be done, this shows a causal link between upper cervical injury and MS and PD patients.

A person with full-spine weakened structure may experience possible sensory, muscular, and circulation problems in all extremities, as well as possible symptoms in heart and lungs, immune weakness, reduced energy levels, pelvic organ problems, urinary, digestive, blood sugar, and blood pressure problems, reproductive, colon issues, autoimmune diseases, thyroid problems, and much more.

When the spinal cord is subjected to stress from postural, structural distortions, your immune system may be affected.[14] Your immune system protects you from disease. With a weakened and distorted spinal structure, the injured nervous system may have a role in immune system effectiveness, leaving you susceptible to many diseases, some life-threatening. A healthy spine and nervous system appear to be closely connected to a healthy immune system.[14]

The nervous system and the immune system have such a multitude of connections that they could correctly be referred to as a single system. The nervous system senses damage, infectious agents, and foreign bodies with the help of chemical-releasing immune cells and deals with these problems by deploying different types of immune cells to carry out specific procedures. Disturbances in the nervous system (subluxations) diminish the ability of an individual to sense and repair damage and combat infection, cancer, etc. directly, resulting in diminished health.[15]

---

[14] http://www.princetonchiropractic.com/papers/publishedImmunestudy.pdf

[15] The Lancet (June 2, 2001). Immunology, An Overview of the Immune System. The Lancet, 357, pp. 1777-1789.

According to "Immunology, An Overview of the Immune System," an article in the medical journal The Lancet:

> *It is becoming clear that the immune system does not work in isolation, but has close communications with other tissues. The interaction of the immune cells with the neurological [spinal cord and nerves] and endocrine systems is now documented.*[16]

> *When the sympathetic nervous system—that part of the autonomic nervous system that works when we are under stress—is over-stimulated from the effect of a distorted posture and weakened curves of the spine, causing stress and tension to the spinal cord, "the activity of the immune system decreases with a resultant increased susceptibility to infection," write Liss and Rabin in an article, "Stress, in the Immune Function and Health," which appeared in The Connection.*[17]

Again, decreased function of the immune system leading to infection also leaves us susceptible to all disease.

---

[16] The Lancet (June 2, 2001). Immunology, An Overview of the Immune System. The Lancet, 357, pp. 1777-1789.

[17] Liss, W., & Rabin, B. (1999). Stress, Immune Function and Health: the Connection. *Stress and Health*, 15:4, pp. 260.

Korr, in 1979 in The Journal of American Osteopath Association, claimed that compromised spinal function (postural and structural weakness of the spine) increases sympathetic tone, the stress response of nerves. Increased and sustained sympathetic tone is linked to immune dysfunction, pain, circulatory dysfunction, progressive nerve dysfunction, and overall reduced health.

Medical research has shown for decades that a distorted, weakened, and injured spinal structure affects the delicate spinal cord, which may weaken overall health.

Unfortunately, some people with poor posture and distorted spinal curves may have no symptoms at all, or may discount minor symptoms as "normal" signs of aging. Your energy level begins to decline. Your immune system gradually weakens. You develop symptoms in your organs, yet they may not seem bad counter drugs seem to calm the symptoms.

The truth is many of the drugs people consume merely cover the symptoms as the disease process progresses in your body. Many of us believe that if we don't feel it, it must be okay, as we race through life busier than ever. Discounted symptoms will continue to progress into disease and eventually a health crisis because the cause of disease has not been addressed.

A paper from the World Health Education Initiative finds:

> *America's healthcare-system-induced deaths are the third leading cause of death in the U.S., after heart disease and cancer. By citing these statistics, Starfield (2000) highlights the need to examine the type of healthcare provided to the U.S. population. The traditional medical paradigm that emphasizes the use of prescription medicine and medical treatment has not only failed to improve the health of Americans, but also led to the decline in the overall well-being of Americans.*[18]

There are many known options for health care choices. We live in an information age where a plethora of information and choices to recover your health are at your fingertips. You can begin to make more empowered choices now that you are becoming aware of the relationship between the nervous and immune systems and the effect of misalignment on nervous system energy flow.

---

[18] Starfield, B. (2000). America's Healthcare System is the Third Leading Cause of Death. World Health Education Initiative. http://www.health-care-reform.net/causedeath.htm

◇◇◇◇◇◇◇◇◇◇◇◇◇◇◇◇◇◇◇◇◇◇

HYPERKYPHOSIS AND FORWARD HEAD POSTURE

...

A forward head posture or position has become a common posture among many people as they age. It's a forward head shift with rounded shoulders, increased forward-bending curve in the mid-back, and a flattened low back. This is also a typical posture of people who sit for long periods (such as people with desk jobs) or who spend prolonged amounts of time looking down at cellphones or tablets.

Here is a side view of possible distorted, injured postures.

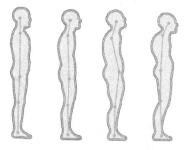

If you follow the red lines from the feet upward, you can see the distortions and "subluxated" regions (regions of the spine out of their normal postural and structural alignment) in the side posture.

The more forward the head shifts, the more the shoulders round, the mid back distorts, the more the low back flattens, the more weight and pressure collapses under the sustained forces of gravity. These are all very dangerous postures, and very common. All are very weak structures geometrically and may collapse or break down quickly, or quicker than they would otherwise.

To your body these weakened, injured postures feel like holding a bowling ball outward with extended arms. The further you extend your arms holding a bowling ball, the heavier the bowling ball feels, the faster you get tired, and the weaker you become until you can no longer hold it up. Basically, you fail because gravity, a force you cannot change, is breaking down your body, posture, spinal cord and health. The more forward your body distorts, the weaker you become. This type of posture also causes great tension and stress on the spinal cord, possibly leading to more severe health problems.

Martin Jungmann, in an article on backaches and posture, writes:

If we regard posture as the result of the dynamic interaction of two factors, the environmental force of gravity on one hand, and the strength of the individual on the other, then posture is but the formal expression of the balance of power existing at any time between the two groups of forces. Thus, any deterioration of the posture indicates that the individual is losing ground in the contest with the environmental forces of gravity.[19]

Gravity always wins, but only if you let it. As the discs between the vertebrae begin to breakdown and degenerate, the openings between the vertebrae, called the intervertebral foramen (the opening where the nerves pass, exiting the spine from the spinal cord to the organs) become reduced.

As a result, there is less room for the nerves to pass freely between the vertebrae. The nerves become compressed, smashed and injured. The organs at the end of those nerves may likely become weak and sick. Losing disc height is very damaging to your health. Degenerative discs from prolonged postural and structural weakness and distortion of the spine can have life-determining effects.

[19] Jungmann, M. (1963). Backaches, Postural Decline, Aging and Gravity-Stain.

J.T. Freeman, M.D., writing in 1957 in the Journal of American Medical Association, says:

Clinical impressions suggest an affirmative answer. Better-postured individuals have fewer defects, enjoy better health, and live longer than those with a seriously distorted skeleton. In general, there is a correlation in body structure, health, and span of survival.[20]

Discs degenerate far earlier than do other musculoskeletal tissues; the first unequivocal findings of degeneration in the lumbar discs are seen in the age group 11–16 years. About 20% of people in their teens have discs with mild signs of degeneration; degeneration increases steeply with age, particularly in males, so that around 10% of 50-year-old discs and 60% of 70-year-old discs are severely degenerate.[21]

Older men with severe disc degeneration have greater AAC (Abdominal Aortic Calcification) severity, faster AAC progression, and higher all-cause mortality rates.[22]

20   Freeman, J.T. (1957). Postural and Health: A Scientific Connection? Posture in the aging and aged body. JAMA, Oct. 19, pp. 843-846.

21   Urban, J. & Roberts, S. (2003). Degeneration of the intervertebral disc. Arthritis Research & Therapy. 5:3, pp. 120-130.

22   Estublier, C., Chapurlat, R., & Szulc, P. (2015). Association of severe disc degeneration with all-cause mortality and abdominal aortic calcification assessed prospectively in older men: findings of a single-center prospective study of osteoporosis in men. Arthritis Rheumatol, 67:5, pp. 1295-304. doi: 10.1002/art.39055

The relationship between spinal and postural distortions and overall quality of health and span of life has been known for 60 years. Again, why haven't we been told by medicine?

In this technology age, young people are being subjected to prolonged forward head and flexion-oriented postures from growing up immersed in the habits of technology and are showing degenerative changes in teenage years similar to adults in their 40's and 50's.

In the past, kids were out playing in the woods, running around on playgrounds, climbing trees—being physical. Parent couldn't keep us inside. Today, at times, we almost insist our kids get outside, and we restrict their technology so they can have a more well-rounded, healthier life. Those families with kids in sports and outside activities will lessen the forward flexion types of postures and accelerated degenerative changes in their child's spine from long hours of flexion distorted postures as they play endless games more than those who don't limit technology time.

Because of these prolonged and sustained forward postures, we are seeing spinal degenerative disorders and health problems in teenagers and young adults that used to be more common in older people. Technology is moving our health into disease and disability.

This also means these same habits will be wreaking havoc on the health and strength of adults who are immersed in these habits and have already developed subluxated, forward-flexed spines. These habits compound and accelerate the degenerative processes of our bodies.

In these forward-flexed postures, discs are under constant abnormal biomechanical stress (again, think of putting your hand on one end of a water balloon). When you press on one side of the water balloon, it displaces out and away from your hand, bulging to the other unweighted side. A disc is similar. Forward-flexed postures place much stress on the front of the discs, forcing them to bulge out the back. Constant compression on the front of the disc, causing it to continually bulge and displace backward, can wear it out very fast, even cause it to bulge and eventually blow out backwards like a flat tire. The spinal cord is behind the disc, so when the disc bulges or herniates and the jelly in the middle of the disc is pushed out of the center of the disc backward into the vulnerable, sensitive spinal cord you become quickly, almost instantaneously disabled. This is analogous to smashing one side of a jelly doughnut. The jelly center gets pushed out. Depending on the extent of the injury and amount of disc "jelly" against the cord and in the spinal canal, surgery is almost inevitable.

Every time your back is stiff or sore and you ignore your weakened spinal structure, you're setting yourself up for an unexpected crisis, whether it be a disc injury, disability, or disease.

I say this because of the thousands of patients with these types of stories. These are stories of patients that used chiropractic for pain management, rather than the structural corrective and health care system. I personally took care of these types of patients myself who insisted on nothing more than pain relief only to watch them suffer with more severe consequences short and long term. I have also heard and seen see these types of patients from the hundreds of chiropractors I have coached. There are plenty of studies showing that abnormal spinal structure leads to chronic pain, disc injury, and eventually to disability, disease, and even early death.[23]

A recent article on spine health said, "All measures of health status showed significantly poorer scores as C7 plumb line deviation increased."[24] This means that the more forward your head and neck are on your shoulders, and the more

23   Kado, D., Li-Yung, L., Ensrud, K., Fink, H., Karlamangla, A., Cummings, S. (2009). Hyperkyphosis predicts mortality independent of vertebral osteoporosis in older women. Study of Osteoporotic Fractures. Nov 19 2009, Ann Intern Med. 2209 May 19, 150(10), pp. 681-687. https://www.ncbi.nlm.nih.gov/pmc/articles/PMC2711520/

24   Glassman, S.D., Bridwell, K., Dimar, J.R., Horton, W., Berven, S., & Schwab, F. (2005). The impact of positive Sagittal balance in Adult Deformity. Spine, 30:18, pp. 2024-2029.

forward-bent your thoracic (rib) cage is, the sicker you will be. In other words, the more forward bent your posture, the worse your health and the shorter your life span.

There are a few variations of this posture. You can't have a problem in one area of the spine without having one in another area of the spine. The spine isn't 3-4 separate regions, but rather one continuous structure from your tailbone to skull. The whole spine always works together from front to side and top to bottom. You always have a full-spine problem, as the spine works as one unit.

An article in Spine magazine found, "Patients with relative kyphosis in the lumbar region (reversal of the normal low back curve) had significantly more disability than patients with normal or lordotic lumbar (normal low back curve) sagittal Cobb measures (side lumbar curve measurement)."[25]

This means that this weakened posture, loss of the normal curves that provide strength and health to the body, creates chronic pain that may likely lead to disability. Have you noticed when you travel there are people on the plane who need wheelchairs? Have you ever noticed their posture? Notice that almost all of them have a bent-forward posture. This is one reason why they are in a wheelchair. Their bodies are weak and disabled. I'm sure if you knew their health

25   Glassman, S.D. et al. (2005). The impact of positive sagittal balance in adult spinal deformity. Spine, 30:18, pp. 2024-2029.

history it would be consistent as well. This truth is all around us and we see it every day. Maybe you will notice it now.

Not knowing this, going to a chiropractor for an adjustment to get rid of back, mid-back or neck pain without correcting the whole structure is like putting a butterfly bandage on a wound that needs 140 stitches. An adjustment may feel good now, while the weakened structure is breaking down, moving you into eventual or sudden disability and disease.

Hyperkyphotic, rounded shoulders and increased curve in the thoracic (mid-back) spine, many times accompanied with a forward head posture, weaken spinal structure, causes stretching and tension stress on the spinal cord. This will not correct on its own. This weakened structure, as shown from the side view in the posture to the far right on page 49, will only collapse. It happens no other way. Gravity always wins, and the spinal cord, the vessel for delivering healing energy in the body, causes the person with this condition to move into loss of function, disease, and possibly premature death.

Here are some comments from an article in the Journal of the American Geriatric Society, "Hyperkyphotic Posture Predicts Mortality in Older Community-Dwelling Men and Women: A Prospective Study":

In age and sex adjusted analysis, persons with hyperkyphotic (increased thoracic curve) posture had a 1.44 (44%) greater rate of mortality.

With increasing kyphotic posture, there was a trend towards greater mortality. Furthermore, even at this mild degree of hyperkyphotic posture, there was a definite greater rate of earlier mortality.[26]

26 Kado, D., Huang, M.H., Karlamangla, A.S., Barrett-Conner, E., & Greendale, G.A. (2004). Hyperkyphotic Posture Predicts Mortality in Older Community-Dwelling Men and Women: A Prospective Study. Journal of the American Geriatric Society. 52:10, pp. 1662.

◇◇◇◇◇◇◇◇◇◇◇◇◇◇◇◇◇◇◇◇◇

HEALTH EFFECTS WITH MINOR SPINAL INJURIES

. . .

Not only can this very weak, sick posture not resist the sustained forces of gravity over time, as discussed, any weakened structure cannot withstand any other force placed onto the spine, even if the force is minor, without a biomechanically detrimental injury of a higher magnitude.

That is, weakened spinal structures, distorted postures, will have less resistance to trauma, and minor incidents may create more impactful, damaging spinal injuries and health problems.

Minor forces may include slips, falls, bumps, abnormal sleeping positions, or athletic injuries. This is similar to attempting to hammer a bent nail into a piece of wood. The nail collapses, even with small strikes of a hammer. Small traumas cause significantly greater damage. Again, the greater the damage, the greater the health problems.

Subluxations of the individual vertebrae or whole curves, especially those complicated by soft-tissue injury, accelerate degeneration, lead to disability, and are known causes of morbidity.[27] [28]

This means that a spine subjected to an outside trauma will have more soft-tissue (ligament and disc) injury, leading to faster degeneration, disability, or even early death. This means you may lose strength and ability to do your daily activities. Your overall function and the health of your body could decline into the state of disease, leading to accelerated aging and premature death.

Your body will weaken progressively faster when your spine has been traumatized causing even minor injury to your spinal cord, than if there was no trauma, or your spinal structure was strong. Injury to your spinal cord includes the physical stress the spinal cord must continually endure due to a weakened spinal structure or abnormal curves from a spinal column that has sustained a trauma.

27   Marchiori, D.M., & Henderson, C.N.R. (1996). A cross-section study correlating cervical radiographic degenerative findings to pain and disability. Spine, 21, pp. 2747-2752.

28   Norris, S.H., & Watt, I. (1983). The prognosis of neck injuries resulting from rear-end collisions. Journal of House and Joint Surgery. 65:B, pp. 608-611.

Again, these traumas originate from anything from sports injuries to minor car accidents, slips, falls, overexertion, prolonged postural strain from desk jobs, or even forward-flexed postures from smart phone use. All of these can cause your health to break down faster and can lead to disease and early death.

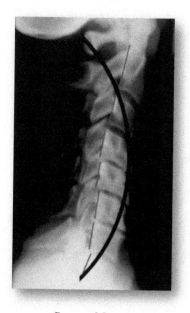 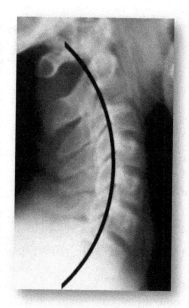

Reversed Curve   *Normal Curve (Lordosis)*

The X-ray on the left shows a weakened structure from trauma with the middle segments, C4 & C5, have been displaced from abnormal compression from weakened, distorted curves and secondary to a whiplash or compressive trauma, like landing on your head. This type of injury is what the research shows will lead to disability and a known cause of morbidity.

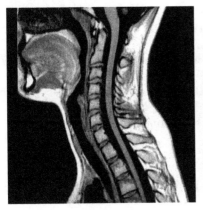 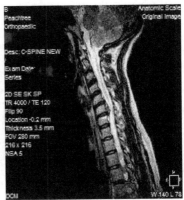

From the side, the normal C-Curve (lordosis) on the left is a strong structure that is resilient to gravity and some trauma. The spinal cord is also very relaxed inside this structure, with no pressure or contact with the spinal canal bringing life-force energy to the organs of the body. The MRI on the right shows a damaged and reversed, kyphotic curve, with the spinal cord in direct physical contact with the spine. This will damage the spinal cord, reduce the energy through the cord to your organs, create disability, form calluses on the cord and may lead to premature death. This MRI may bring a more clear reality to the importance of spinal structure to strength and health for life.

An article in the Journal of Spinal Disorders & Techniques says,

Maintaining normal cervical anatomy with its lordosis in this region of prominent movement may optimize the cord function. [29]

29   Ozer, E., Yuccsoy, K., Yurstever, C., Secil, M. (2007). Kyphosis One Level Above the Cervical Disc Disease: Is the kyphosis Cause or Effect? Journal of Spinal Disorders & Techniques, 20:1, pp. 14-19. Departments of Neurosurgery and Radiology. Dokuz Eylul University: Izmir, Turkey.

An abnormality or distortion of the curves causes the spine to lose its resiliency and shock-absorbing qualities, which leads to further compression, weakness, and susceptibility to trauma and breakdown. These normal, healthy spinal curves from the side give us the ability to withstand compression because they give our structure its spring-like qualities, as the force of compression is distributed along the whole curve. This quality is called *radially loading*. The force is spread through the whole arc. This is a principle of physics and is used to build dams that hold back the force of rivers, the arc in a bridge that supports the weight of cars and trucks and more.

Loss of the normal cervical curve from the side can collapse into a forward-bending, weakened posture as it progressively spreads downward into the thoracic spine. We are seeing this more at younger ages as teenagers carry heavy backpacks to school and use cellphones and tech devices.

Minor traumas can cause weaknesses that create an unstable structure. As the injured spinal structure progressively weakens, the other curves can break down, and the collapsing spine spreads into their mid-back and lower back. This is also one of the reasons why people feel back pain, because the whole spine is collapsing, creating an increased burden on the low back. As their whole spine becomes weak, they lose the ability to walk well because they have lost their ability and strength to move—they are "disabled." They must use oxygen tanks because the forward-distorted posture with forward-bending, hunched upper back and forward head can affect lung function.[30]

> Worsening spinal deformity is associated with deteriorating lung function.[31]

> Altered biomechanics in the cervico-thoracic area as well as changes in the muscle force length relationships are important factors that determine respiratory performance.[32]

They have lost their strength and ability to breathe and ambulate, to move in any way.

> Older persons with hyperkyphotic posture are more likely to have physical functional difficulties.[30]

---

[30] Kado et al. (2005). J. Gerontol: A bio. *Science Medical Science*, 60:5, pp. 633-637.

[31] Tattersall, R., & Walshall, M.J. (2003). JR Soc Med, 96:18.

[32] Kapreli, E. et al. (2009). Respiratory Dysfunction in chronic neck pain patients: pilot study. Posture and Cystic Fibrosis Cephalpgia, 29, 701-710.

Increased pain in cervical and lumbar spine-related increased FP

(forward posture of the body). Also depression, motivation, muscle

impairment, balance, gait and Disability scores.[33]

Gravity, over time, has completely broken down their physical strength and organs due to a weakened spinal structure and stretched, stressed, and tensed spinal cord.

33
51, pp. 1419-1426.   Balzini, L. et al. (2003). Hyper-Kyphosis & +TzH. American Geriatric Society,

◇◇◇◇◇◇◇◇◇◇◇◇◇◇◇◇◇◇◇◇

DANGERS OF FORWARD-FLEXED HEAD AND NECK POSTURES

...

L et's look at the health effects of losing your cervical curve.

This is especially important because your neck is just under your skull, which houses the brain. Optimal nerve function in your neck is crucial because spinal cord stress in your neck will cause whole body, systemic disease. You can lose your normal curve with trauma (almost everyone has experienced some form of minor or major whiplash injury). As I've mentioned, you can lose the normal cervical curve from extended and prolonged postural positions like bending your head forward when you look down at your phone, work at a computer, lie on the couch with your chin toward your chest, or even when sleeping on two pillows.

This applies to any posture that involves putting your head forward with your chin approaching your chest. When the spine bends forward, the spinal cord is forced to follow the spine. Therefore, it is forced to stretch like an overstretched rubber band to fit into that weakened, distorted structure.

Here is an illustration of a normal, relaxed spinal cord with a normal cervical curve radiograph.

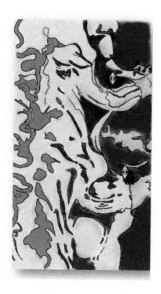 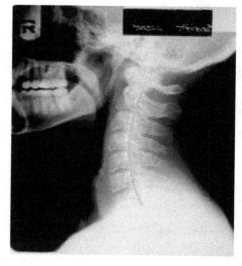

The illustration on the left shows a slackened cord, rich with blood flow. This X-ray on the right is representative of a normal cervical curve, or *lordosis*. On the left, you see that a slackened, relaxed spinal cord is like a powerline delivering proper life-force energy in the form of electrical impulses down the spine and into every organ and cell in the body. This is typical of a spinal cord within a normal cervical curve.

Next is an illustration of an overstretched cord from a loss of cervical curve, most commonly from a forward head posture or loss of the normal cervical lordosis.

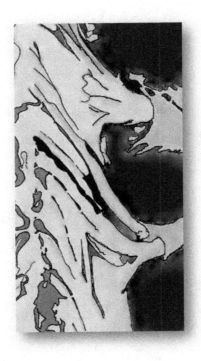

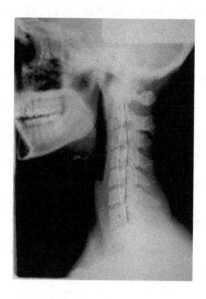

This spinal cord must stretch due to the reversal (kyphosis) of the normal curve.

When the curve is lost or reverses, the intra-cord pressure increases from tension in the cord, the diameter decreases, and it ceases to provide the needed energy for health. When an electrical cord is under abnormal tension it reduces the conductivity of the cord. This is true of the spinal cord.

The increased tension in the cord also diminishes blood flow in the cord. As you may already know, reduced blood flow to any tissue in the body reduces nutrients and oxygen, and begins to break down that tissue and cause it to die. When your spinal cord begins to lose blood flow and die, you shut down the energy to all functions in your body. When your spinal cord dies, *you* die!

Energy keeping the body healthy flows from the brain through the spinal cord into the organs. With forward-flexed neck postures, such as bending forward looking at your cellphone, the cord displaces forward, pressing against the back of the vertebrae, in physical contact with the bony structure. After 10 minutes of such a sustained posture, the ligaments of the spine begin to deform and change into this abnormal structure.

This process is called plastic deformation. Plastic deformation creates more permanent change in the length of the ligaments. The ligaments will take on the form of your sustained posture and spinal position. This causes sustained stress and tension in the spinal cord as the spine deforms into that structure.

> *Progressive kyphosis of the cervical spine (reversal of the cervical curve) resulted in demyelination (breakdown of the fatty covering of the nerves and cord that conducts electrical impulses along the nerves/cord) of the nerve fibers...due to chronic compression of the spinal cord.*[34]

[34] Shimizu, K., Nakamura, M., Nishikawa, Y., Hijikata, S., Chiba, K., & Toyama, Y. (2005). Spinal Kyphosis Causes Demyelination and Neuronal Loss in the Spinal Cord: A New Model of Kyphotic Deformity. Spine, 30:210, pp. 2388-2392.

Again, as stated earlier, demyelination of the cord leads to breakdown of the cord, paralysis, and loss of function of organs. Diseases like Multiple Sclerosis and ALS are examples of demyelinating diseases.

> *Loss of lordosis or kyphotic alignment of the cervical spine and spinal cord may contribute to the development of myelopathy and in patients with cervical kyphotic deformity, the spinal cord could be compressed by tethering over the apical vertebrae or the intervertebral disc.*[35]

In other words, when the neck loses its normal C-Curve to become straight, or progresses until it reverses and curves backwards, the spinal cord will get smashed and stretched against the vertebrae where the spine kinks in the opposite direction, like bending a garden hose around a corner of a wall. The example is on page 62.

The kink in the spine also causes compression on the disc, pushing it back into the spinal cord. The result is a smashed spinal cord, which means loss of function. Since we are talking about the neck, this condition weakens the rest of your body, everything below that injury, your whole body. This is the result of prolonged forward-bending postures and traumas to the cervical spine.

We conclude that the (cervical spine) sagittal kyphotic deformity related to flexion mechanical stress may be a significant factor in the development of cervical spondylotic myelopathy(sustained flexion forward-bending of the neck increases cord stretching and tension), and seems to be closely associated with the resultant increase in the anterior compressive effect on the spinal cord.[35]

When the spinal cord is being stretched (longitudinal stress) and the front of the cord is being smashed against the vertebrae, you will lose motor function. At the same time, the back of the spinal cord is being stretched, which also reduces nerve flow. The front of the cord is being smashed, and the back is being stretched. The back of the cord is where the sensory nerve tracts are located. You could potentially be losing motor function from the front of the cord and sensory function from stretching of the back of the cord. That really means your body is getting weaker and you can't feel it.

35   Kenzo, U., Hideaki, N., Ryuichiro, S., Takafum, I.Y., Erisa, S.M., Shigeru, K., & Hisatoshi, B. (2009). Cervical Spondylotic Myelopathy Associated with Kyphosis or Sagittal Sigmoid Alignment: Outcome After Anterior or Posterior Decompression. Journal of Neurosurgery: Spine, 11, pp. 521-528.

Cervical pathology, mediated through sympathetic nerves, has been associated with a number of disorders, which include about 20 kinds of diseases or symptom groups, such as hypertension, cardiac arrhythmias, dizziness, eyesight malfunction and gastrointestinal dysfunction.[36]

Twenty types of diseases are, truthfully, only the beginning. A weakened immune system leaves you vulnerable to any type of disease. Signs of a weakened immune system range from the common cold and flu to cancer, from a sniffle to a life-threatening disease.

To increase the likelihood of a long, healthy, functional, and strong life, you must address, correct, and maintain your spinal structure and nervous system, and know how to use your body in a healthy manner. Research says your life is dependent on this fact.

It is not necessary to do this if you don't care. It is mandatory if you do. Now you know what hasn't been told to you by your medical doctor. It's not all the MD's fault. Medical doctors are taught by the companies that infiltrate and determine their curriculum in medical school, by pharmaceutical companies, who are in the business to sell you drugs, not keep you healthy. If this were common knowledge

---

[36] Song, X.H., Xu, X.X., Ding, L.W., Cao, L., Sadel, A., & Wen, H. (2007). A Preliminary Study of Neck-Stomach Syndrome. *World Journal of Gastroenterology*, 13:18, pp. 2575-2580.

what would happen to the sale of drugs and the profits of disease in this capitalistic health care system? That means power belongs to those with the most money. Do you trust a system that is ruled by multi-billion dollar organizations that profit from your disease?

Your health is your responsibility. This book is in your hands because you are taking responsibility to make informed, empowering decisions for yourself, for your family and for those whom you care about who will listen.

Your spinal structure dictates the function of your nervous system, which controls your overall health—an understanding that has always been known, but has, in our technologically driven society, become severely neglected, under communicated, and often overlooked, even hidden. Ancient civilizations have put these principles into practice for centuries. Americans are now becoming aware of what other civilizations and societies have practiced since their inception thousands of years ago.

This is not a new principle, but an old one. This book gives you a new opportunity for better health.

The next question is, "What do you do?"

◇◇◇◇◇◇◇◇◇◇◇◇◇◇◇◇◇◇◇◇◇◇◇

THE 5–10s

...

I n 10 minutes of this forward-flexed, sustained posture, your spinal ligaments begin to abnormally deform, to take on the shape of your distorted spine. This means injury to your spine can begin in as little as 10 minutes.

Because of this, I have developed the 5–10s. These are five activities you can do to begin to relieve the stress and strain on your spine and spinal cord to give you some temporary activities to relieve stress and renew your health. The first four 10s are very temporary relief and should be done every day. The fifth 10 is for more permanent correction and should be done by everyone who desires to live their life with confidence, strength and freedom with their health. After you notice you have been in a forward, hunched-over posture for at least 10 minutes, you can perform these exercises daily to relieve stress on your body.

1.   <u>10 BACK EXTENSIONS.</u> Stand up with your arms relaxed at your side. Turn your palms out by rotating at your shoulders, not just by turning your hands. In other words, rotate your whole arm at the shoulder by turning your thumbs all the way outward like you are hitchhiking. Now push your chest out, arch your low back by sticking out your belly, and lay your head all the way back. If you begin to feel off balance, do this seated in a chair. Hold this position for 10 seconds, then perform 10 repetitions. You can also support your back if you feel weak or unsupported. When you get stronger, you can perform these while lying down. See the diagram below.

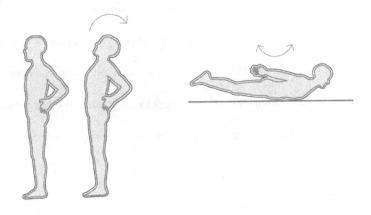

2. 10 DEEP DIAPHRAGMATIC BREATHS. Breathe deeply from your diaphragm. This is not chest breathing. When you breathe, don't raise your chest. When you breathe in, expand your belly, as a baby breathes. This is breathing from your diaphragm. Forward-flexed, hunched posture shuts down deep breathing, so your body is less oxygenated, becoming fatigued and weak. Diaphragmatic breathing brings oxygen into the deepest recesses of your lungs, where true oxygen exchange takes place. Do this deep-breathing exercise as you are doing your back-extension exercise. These should be done together. Perform 10 breaths with your 10 back extensions. Hold each breath for five seconds. You should feel your body energize and come back to life.

3. DRINK WATER IN 10-OUNCE INCREMENTS. You should drink half your body weight in ounces of water every day, in 10-ounce increments. If you weigh 200 pounds, drink 100 ounces of water, or ten 10-ounce glasses per day. Forward-flexed postures compress the discs in your spine and push out the water, which leads to disc degeneration and aging of your body. Disc tissue will hydrate only after your nervous system and organs are hydrated first. That is your body's hydration priority, therefore, you must be fully hydrated to replenish lost water to the disc again. Hydrating with motion in the spine will

replenish the water in the discs and in the organs, and restore healing in your body. Adding decompression/axial traction will help rehydrate discs as long as you are simultaneously doing a spinal corrective program like Chiropractic BioPhysics®.

4. 10 MINUTES ON A ROLLED TOWEL UNDER YOUR NECK AND LOW BACK. Roll a bath towel into a tight roll and use rubber bands to keep it rolled tightly to put under your low back. Then roll a smaller towel tightly using rubber bands to put under your lower neck. Put the low back towel under the base of your low back. Place the neck towel under the top of your shoulders, low on your neck and high on your upper back and shoulders. Lay your head back and be sure the back of your head can touch the floor, while pushing a curve in your cervical spine. If your head can't touch the floor, your towel is too big. Lie on these for 10 minutes or more. This may be very uncomfortable at first. Only lie on these for a limited time if you get sore, and work your way up to over 10 minutes. Do not attempt to push yourself into pain because it may be detrimental in this case. Work up to up 20 minutes. If you are very flexible increase the time to 30 mins. This will help to induce a better curve in your neck and back, relieve stress on the spinal cord, and begin to reshape

the ligaments into a healthier structure. This can be done every day as many times as you need.

5. <u>TAKE 10 MINUTES AND GO TO **CBP PATIENT**</u> (*www.CBPPatient. com*) You can find highly trained doctors in your area who have been trained in the most advanced system of spinal correction available, which can make permanent changes in your spinal structure, giving you a healthy nervous system for a strong, healthy body and life. If no doctors are close to you, it's worth traveling to get an evaluation to the nearest CBP® doctor, if possible. These doctors can also fit you for a Denneroll, an orthotic for your cervical, thoracic and lumbar spine. These spinal orthotics, which you must be tested (with an X-ray) and fitted according to your specific spinal problem. It is made for you to use at home and can assist in more permanent correction of your spine. It's much more powerful to make permanent changes in your spinal structure than using a towel, the fourth exercise in the 5-10s. The towel exercise may temporarily relieve stress and the Denneroll system is for far more predictable correction.

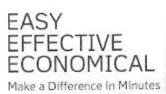

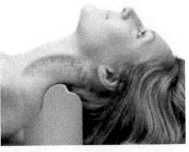

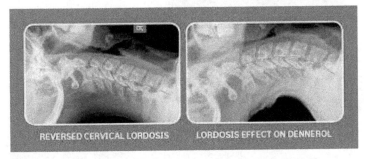

REVERSED CERVICAL LORDOSIS   LORDOSIS EFFECT ON DENNEROL

This picture shows the actual cervical Denneroll. You can see the woman's loss of cervical curve on the left, and you can see how the Denneroll will reshape your spine into a new structure.

If you use this device for the next 90-180 days in combination with treatment, you will see this change in your spinal structure that will change the strength and health of your body for the rest of your life. You can call doctors in your area and ask them if they will test you with a cervical Denneroll. With these 5–10s, anyone can get "back" to health.

◇◇◇◇◇◇◇◇◇◇◇◇◇◇◇◇◇◇◇◇

LIFE PURPOSE

...

I believe most people believe they are here to fulfill some purpose in life. This is the reason this book exists, to help bring awareness, choice, empowerment, and a plan of action to help you and millions 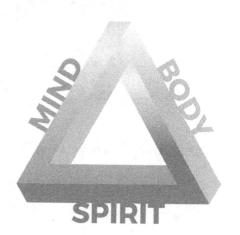 of others live a better, healthier life. This book has life-changing information that may lead to one of the most important decisions in your life and the lives of people you share this book with. I also believe we are here to contribute to the lives of others. First we take care of our health and life, so we can have a greater impact in others. If you believe the same, please share this message and this book. It is my desire to give you confidence in your body and health, freedom to live the life that you desire, and tools to lead others to do the same.

Perform these 5–10s and, most importantly, find a CBP® doctor in your area, and live a healthier, more fulfilling life.

Dr. Fred DiDomenico

About the Author

...

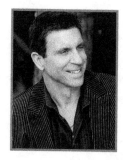

D r. Fred DiDomenico grew up in Southern California. After receiving his degree from Los Angeles College of Chiropractic, he began to specialize in spinal correction. Over the course of 14 years, his practice grew to four spinal-corrective offices, focusing on Chiropractic BioPhysics, and he and his staff helped between 550 and 700 clients a week.

Despite this thriving client base, Dr. Fred wanted to spread the message to a larger public about the benefits of corrective chiropractic. After intense study of human behavior, influential communicators and business principles, Dr. Fred formed Elite Chiropractic Coaching in 2008 to create and advise others to build powerful, relationship-based and self-empowered clinical and business systems that advance the chiropractic profession and that provide a fuller impression of chiropractic to the general public.

For Dr. Fred, spinal correction is the highest, most powerful application of the principles of chiropractic truth, "a health care system and a lifestyle, and chiropractors are self-empowerment coaches who teach people how to take responsibility for their lives and health." He believes that people who are subluxated and suffering from a variety of diseases can heal through the chiropractic principles of an optimal spine, optimal health lifestyle.

This forward-thinking, bold and innovative model has led to a rapid growth in Elite Chiropractic Coaching businesses.

Dr. Fred has appeared on numerous platforms, television and radio, to speak about the effect of technology on the spine and its relationship with disease, as well as on self-empowerment, the principle of chiropractic, the philosophy of chiropractic, and the business principles of communication. He also has his own YouTube channel, where he shares his experiences in teaching and coaching, and reveals new breakthroughs in the field.

This book will reveal to you the foundational cause of chronic pain, disability, disease, and even a shortened life span—a cause that you will not find mentioned on your evening news channel. There is extensive medical research available that supports this information and has been available for decades, yet the release of this information would change the healthcare system—not only in this country, but throughout the world—if it became common knowledge.

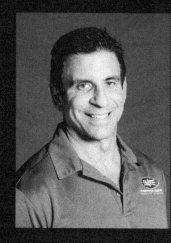

This book will also awaken you to how technologically based daily habits in this advancing world are creating postural and neurological weakness in our spine and nervous system that causes degenerative spinal conditions beginning in children and teenagers and rapidly progressing into adulthood. These are conditions that, in the past, didn't usually present themselves until mid-life or old age. This book also explains how these postural habits are damaging our spinal cords and overall health, leading to the many rapidly-advancing diseases we are seeing today.

To combat this, you will be introduced to the "5-10s." These are 5 exercises and habits that can change the effects of these stresses on your spine and nervous system. You can take back your health! The intention of this book is to give you back control and certainty that you can live an empowered, healthy, rejuvenated life with a strong mind and body. If you want this confidence and freedom, read this book, take action, and give the knowledge to others to help them do the same.

Dr. Fred DiDomenico

CPSIA information can be obtained
at www.ICGtesting.com
Printed in the USA
LVHW042309270323
742785LV00014B/705